THE ANTI STROKE DIET COOKBOOK

GEORGE ANDERSON

CHAPTER ONE

INTRODUCTION

Stroke

A stroke is a medical condition in which poor blood flow to the brain causes cell death. There are two main types of stroke: ischemic, due to lack of blood flow, and hemorrhagic, due to bleeding. Both cause parts of the brain to stop functioning properly.

Signs and symptoms of a stroke may include an inability to move or feel on one side of the body, problems understanding or speaking, dizziness, or loss of vision to one side. Signs and symptoms often appear soon after the stroke has occurred. If symptoms last less than one or two hours, the stroke is a transient ischemic attack (TIA), also called a mini-stroke. A hemorrhagic stroke may also be associated with a severe headache. The symptoms of a stroke can be permanent. Long-term complications may include pneumonia and loss of bladder control.

The main risk factor for stroke is high blood pressure. Other risk factors include high blood cholesterol, tobacco smoking, obesity, diabetes mellitus, a previous TIA, end-stage kidney disease, and atrial fibrillation. An ischemic stroke is typically caused by blockage of a blood vessel, though there are also fewer common causes. A hemorrhagic stroke is caused by either bleeding directly into the brain or into the space between the brain's membranes. Bleeding may occur due to a ruptured brain aneurysm. Diagnosis is typically based on a physical exam and supported by medical imaging such as a CT scan or MRI scan. A CT scan can rule out bleeding, but may not necessarily rule out ischemia, which early on typically does not show up on a CT scan. Other tests such as an electrocardiogram (ECG) and blood tests are done to determine risk factors and rule out other possible causes. Low blood sugar may cause similar symptoms.

Prevention includes decreasing risk factors, surgery to open up the arteries to the brain in those with problematic carotid narrowing, and warfarin in people with atrial fibrillation. Aspirin or statins may be recommended by physicians for prevention. A stroke or TIA often re□uires emergency care. An ischemic stroke, if detected within three to four and half hours, may be treatable with a medication that can break down the clot. Some hemorrhagic strokes benefit from surgery. Treatment to attempt recovery of lost function is called stroke rehabilitation, and ideally takes place in a stroke unit; however, these are not available in much of the world.

In 2013, approximately 6.9 million people had an ischemic stroke and 3.4 million people had a hemorrhagic stroke. In 2015, there were about 42.4 million people who had previously had a stroke and were still alive. Between 1990 and 2010 the number of strokes which occurred each year decreased by approximately 10% in the developed world and increased by 10% in the developing world. In 2015, stroke was the second most frequent cause of death after coronary artery disease, accounting for 6.3 million deaths (11% of the total). About 3.0 million deaths resulted from ischemic stroke while 3.3 million deaths resulted from hemorrhagic stroke. About half of people who have had a stroke live less than one year. Overall, two thirds of strokes occurred in those over 65 years old.

WHAT IS A STROKE?

A stroke occurs when a blood vessel in the brain ruptures and bleeds, or when there's a blockage in the blood supply to the brain. The rupture or blockage prevents blood and oxygen from reaching the brain's tissues.

According to the Centers for Disease Control and Prevention (CDC), stroke is a leading cause of death in the United States. Every year, more than 795,000 U.S. people have a stroke.

Without oxygen, brain cells and tissue become damaged and begin to die within minutes.

There are three primary types of strokes:

• Transient ischemic attack (TIA) involves a blood clot that typically reverses on its own.

• Ischemic stroke involves a blockage caused by either a clot or pla☐ue in the artery. The symptoms and complications of ischemic stroke can last longer than those of a TIA, or may become permanent.

• Hemorrhagic stroke is caused by either a burst or leaking blood vessel that seeps into the brain.

Stroke symptoms

The loss of blood flow to the brain damages tissues within the brain. Symptoms of a stroke show up in the body parts controlled by the damaged areas of the brain.

The sooner a person having a stroke gets care, the better their outcome is likely to be. For this reason, it's helpful to know the signs of a stroke so you can act quickly. Stroke symptoms can include:

• paralysis

• numbness or weakness in the arm, face, and leg, especially on one side of the body

• trouble speaking or understanding others

• slurred speech

• confusion, disorientation, or lack of responsiveness

• sudden behavioral changes, especially increased agitation

• vision problems, such as trouble seeing in one or both eyes with vision blackened or blurred, or double vision

• trouble walking

• loss of balance or coordination

• dizziness

• severe, sudden headache with an unknown cause

• seizures

• nausea or vomiting

A stroke re□uires immediate medical attention. If you think you or someone else is having a stroke, call 911 or local emergency services right away.

Prompt treatment is key to preventing the following outcomes:

• brain damage

• long-term disability

• death

It's better to be overly cautious when dealing with a stroke, so don't be afraid to get emergency medical help if you think you recognize the signs of a stroke.

What causes a stroke?

The cause of a stroke depends on the type of stroke. Strokes fall into three main categories:

• transient ischemic attack (TIA)

• ischemic stroke

• hemorrhagic stroke

These categories can be further broken down into other types of strokes, including:

• embolic stroke

• thrombotic stroke

- intracerebral stroke

- subarachnoid stroke

The type of stroke you have affects your treatment and recovery process.

Ischemic stroke

During an ischemic stroke, the arteries supplying blood to the brain narrow or become blocked. Blood clots or severely reduced blow flow to the brain causes these blockages. Pieces of plaque breaking off and blocking a blood vessel can also cause them.

There are two types of blockages that can lead to ischemic stroke: a cerebral embolism and cerebral thrombosis.

A cerebral embolism (often referred to as embolic stroke) occurs when a blood clot forms in another part of the body often the heart or arteries in the upper chest and neck and moves through the bloodstream until it hits an artery too narrow to let it pass.

The clot gets stuck, and stops the flow of blood and causes a stroke.

Cerebral thrombosis (often referred to as thrombotic stoke) occurs when a blood clot develops at the fatty plaque within the blood vessel.

According to the CDC, 87 percent of strokes are ischemic strokes.

Transient ischemic attack (TIA)

A transient ischemic attack, often called a TIA or ministroke, occurs when blood flow to the brain is blocked temporarily.

Symptoms are similar to those of a full stroke. However, they're typically temporary and disappear after a few minutes or hours, when the blockage moves and blood flow is restored.

A blood clot usually causes a TIA. While it's not technically categorized as a full stroke, a TIA serves as a warning that an actual stroke may happen. Because of this, it's best not to ignore it. Seek the same treatment you would for a major stroke and get emergency medical help.

According to the CDC, more than one-third of people who experience a TIA and don't get treatment have a major stroke within a year. Up to 10 to 15 percent of people who experience a TIA have a major stroke within 3 months.

Hemorrhagic stroke

A hemorrhagic stroke happens when an artery in the brain breaks open or leaks blood. The blood from that artery creates excess pressure in the skull and swells the brain, damaging brain cells and tissues.

The two types of hemorrhagic strokes are intracerebral and subarachnoid:

• An intracerebral hemorrhagic stroke is the most common type of hemorrhagic stroke. It happens when the tissues surrounding the brain fill with blood after an artery bursts.

• A subarachnoid hemorrhagic stroke is less common. It causes bleeding in the area between the brain and the tissues that cover it.

According to the American Heart Association, about 13 percent of strokes are hemorrhagic.

RISK FACTORS FOR STROKE

Certain risk factors make you more susceptible to stroke. According to the National Heart, Lung, and Blood Institute, risk factors for stroke include:

Diet

An unbalanced diet can increase the risk of stroke. This type of diet is high in:

• salt

• saturated fats

• trans fats

• cholesterol

Inactivity

Inactivity, or lack of exercise, can also raise the risk of stroke.

Regular exercise has a number of health benefits. The CDC recommends that adults get at least 2.5 hours of aerobic exercise every week. This can mean simply a brisk walk a few times a week.

Heavy alcohol use

The risk of stroke also increases with heavy alcohol use.

If you drink, drink in moderation. This means no more than one drink a day for women, and no more than two drinks a day for men.

Heavy alcohol use can raise blood pressure levels. It can also raise triglyceride levels, which can cause atherosclerosis. This is plaque buildup in the arteries that narrows blood vessels.

Tobacco use

Using tobacco in any form also raises the risk of stroke, since it can damage the blood vessels and heart. Nicotine also raises blood pressure.

Personal background

There are some risk factors for stroke you can't control, such as:

• Family history. Stroke risk is higher in some families because of genetic health factors, such as high blood pressure.

• Sex. According to the CDC, while both women and men can have strokes, they're more common in women than in men in all age groups.

• Age. The older you are, the more likely you are to have a stroke.

• Race and ethnicity. African Americans, Alaska Natives, and American Indians are more likely to have a stroke than other racial groups.

Health history

Certain medical conditions are linked to stroke risk. These include:

• a previous stroke or TIA

• high blood pressure

• high cholesterol

• carrying too much excess weight

• heart disorders, such as coronary artery disease

• heart valve defects

• enlarged heart chambers and irregular heartbeats

• sickle cell disease

• diabetes

• blood clotting disorder

• patent foramen ovale (PFO)

To find out about your specific risk factors for stroke, talk with your doctor.

Complications

The complications after stroke can vary. They may occur because of either a direct injury to the brain during the stroke, or because abilities have been permanently affected.

Some of these complications include:

- seizures

- loss of bladder and bowel control

- cognitive impairment, including dementia

- reduced mobility, range of motion, or ability to control certain muscle movements

- depression

- mood or emotional changes

- shoulder pain

- bed sores

- sensory or sensation changes

These complications can be managed by methods such as:

- medication

- physical therapy

- counseling

Certain complications may even be reserved.

How to prevent a stroke

Lifestyle changes can't prevent all strokes. But many of these changes can make a radical difference when it comes to lowering your risk of stroke.

These changes include the following:

• Quit smoking. If you smoke, quitting now will lower your risk of stroke. You can reach out to your doctor to create a quit plan.

• Limit alcohol use. Heavy alcohol consumption can raise your blood pressure, which in turn raises the risk of stroke. If reducing your intake is difficult, reach out to your doctor for help.

• Keep a moderate weight. Overweight and obesity increases the risk of stroke. To help manage your weight, eat a balanced diet and stay physically active more often than not. Both steps can also reduce blood pressure and cholesterol levels.

• Get regular checkups. Talk with your doctor about how often to get a checkup for blood pressure, cholesterol, and any conditions you may have. They can also support you in making these lifestyle changes and offer guidance.

Taking all these measures will help put you in better shape to prevent stroke.

DIAGNOSIS OF STROKE

Your doctor will ask you or a family member about your symptoms and what you were doing when they arose. They'll take your medical history to find out your stroke risk factors. They'll also:

• ask what medications you take

• check your blood pressure

• listen to your heart

You'll also have a physical exam, during which your doctor will evaluate you for:

• balance

• coordination

• weakness

• numbness in your arms, face, or legs

• signs of confusion

• vision issues

Your doctor will then do certain tests to help confirm a stroke diagnosis. These tests can help them determine whether you had a stroke and, if so:

• what may have caused it

• what part of the brain is affected

• whether you have bleeding in the brain

Tests to diagnose stroke

Your doctor may order various tests to further help them determine whether you've had a stroke, or to rule out another condition. These tests include:

Blood tests

Your doctor might draw blood for several blood tests. Blood tests can determine:

• blood sugar levels

• whether you have an infection

• platelet counts

• how fast your blood clots

• cholesterol levels

MRI and CT scan

Your doctor may order may an MRI scan, CT scan, or both.

An MRI can help see whether any brain tissue or brain cells have been damaged.

A CT scan can provide a detailed and clear picture of your brain, which can show any bleeding or damage. It may also show other brain conditions that could be causing your symptoms.

EKG

An electrocardiogram (EKG) is a simple test that records the electrical activity in the heart, measuring its rhythm and recording how fast it beats.

An EKG can determine whether you have any heart conditions that may have led to a stroke, such as a prior heart attack or atrial fibrillation.

Cerebral angiogram

A cerebral angiogram offers a detailed look at the arteries in your neck and brain. The test can show blockages or clots that may have caused symptoms.

Carotid ultrasound

A carotid ultrasound, also called a carotid duplex scan, can show fatty deposits (plaque) in your carotid arteries, which supply the blood to your face, neck, and brain.

It can also show whether your carotid arteries have been narrowed or blocked.

Echocardiogram

An echocardiogram can find sources of clots in your heart. These clots may have traveled to your brain and caused a stroke.

CHAPTER TWO

STROKE TREATMENT

Proper medical evaluation and prompt treatment are vital to recovering from a stroke. According to the American Heart Association and American Stroke Association, "Time lost is brain lost."

Call 911 or local emergency services as soon as you realize you may be having a stroke, or if you suspect someone else is having a stroke.

Treatment for stroke depends on the type of stroke:

Ischemic stroke and TIA

Since a blood clot or blockage in the brain causes these stroke types, they're largely treated with similar techniques. They can include:

Clot-breaking drugs

Thrombolytic drugs can break up blood clots in your brain's arteries, which will stop the stroke and reduce damage to the brain.

One such drug, tissue plasminogen activator (tPA), or Alteplase IV r-tPA, is considered the gold standard in ischemic stroke treatment.

This drug works by dissolving blood clots ꓪuickly.

People who receive a tPA injection are more likely to recover from a stroke and less likely to have any lasting disability as a result of the stroke.

Mechanical thrombectomy

During this procedure, a doctor inserts a catheter into a large blood vessel inside your head. They then use a device to pull the clot out of the vessel. This surgery is most successful if it's performed 6 to 24 hours after the stroke begins.

Stents

If a doctor finds where artery walls have weakened, they may perform a procedure to inflate the narrowed artery and support the walls of the artery with a stent.

Surgery

In the rare instances that other treatments don't work, surgery can remove a blood clot and plaques from your arteries.

This surgery may be done with a catheter. If the clot is especially large, a surgeon may open an artery to remove the blockage.

Hemorrhagic stroke

Strokes caused by bleeds or leaks in the brain require different treatment strategies. Treatments for hemorrhagic stroke include:

Medications

Unlike with an ischemic stroke, if you're having a hemorrhagic stroke, the treatment goal is to make your blood clot. Therefore, you may be given medication to counteract any blood thinners you take.

You may also be prescribed drugs that can:

• reduce blood pressure

- lower the pressure in your brain

- prevent seizures

- prevent blood vessel constriction

Coiling

During this procedure, your doctor guides a long tube to the area of hemorrhage or weakened blood vessel. They then install a coil-like device in the area where the artery wall is weak. This blocks blood flow to the area, reducing bleeding.

Clamping

During imaging tests, your doctor may discover an aneurysm that hasn't started bleeding yet or has stopped.

To prevent additional bleeding, a surgeon may place a tiny clamp at the base of the aneurysm. This cuts off blood supply and prevents a possible broken blood vessel or new bleeding.

Surgery

If your doctor sees that an aneurysm has burst, they may do surgery to clip the aneurysm and prevent additional bleeding. Likewise, a craniotomy may be needed to relieve the pressure on the brain after a large stroke.

In addition to emergency treatment, your healthcare team will advise you on ways to prevent future strokes.

Stroke medications

Several medications are used to treat strokes. The type your doctor prescribes depends largely on the type of stroke you had.

The goal of some medications is to prevent a second stroke, while others aim to prevent a stroke from happening in the first place.

Your doctor may prescribe one or more of these medications to treat or prevent a stroke, depending on factors such as your health history and your risks.

The most common stroke medications include:

Direct-acting oral anticoagulants (DOACs)

This newer drug class works in the same way as traditional anticoagulants (reducing your blood's ability to clot), but they often work faster and require less monitoring.

If taken for stroke prevention, DOACs may also reduce the risk of brain bleed.

Tissue plasminogen activator (tPA)

This emergency medication can be given during a stroke to break up the blood clot causing the stroke. It's the only medication currently available that can do this, but it must be given within 3 to 4.5 hours after symptoms of a stroke begin.

This drug is injected into a blood vessel so the medication can start to work as □uickly as possible, which reduces the risk of complications from the stroke.

Anticoagulants

These drugs reduce your blood's ability to clot. The most common anticoagulant is warfarin (Coumadin, Jantoven).

These drugs can also prevent existing blood clots from growing larger, which is why doctors may prescribe them to prevent a stroke, or after an ischemic stroke or TIA has occurred.

Antiplatelet drugs

These medications prevent blood clots by making it more difficult for the blood's platelets to stick together. The most common antiplatelet drugs include aspirin and clopidogrel (Plavix).

The drugs can prevent ischemic strokes. They're especially important in preventing secondary stroke.

If you've never had a stroke before, only use aspirin as a preventive medication if you have a high risk of atherosclerotic cardiovascular disease (e.g., heart attack and stroke) and a low risk of bleeding.

Statins

Statins help lower high blood cholesterol levels. They're among the most commonly prescribed medications in the United States.

These drugs prevent the production of an enzyme that can turn cholesterol into plaque the thick, sticky substance that can build up on the walls of arteries and cause strokes and heart attacks.

Common statins include:

• rosuvastatin (Crestor)

• simvastatin (Zocor)

• atorvastatin (Lipitor)

Blood pressure drugs

High blood pressure can cause pieces of plaque buildup in your arteries to break off. These pieces can block arteries, causing a stroke.

As a result, managing high blood pressure with medication, lifestyle changes, or both can help prevent a stroke.

Recovering from a stroke

Stroke is a leading cause of long-term disability in the United States.

However, the American Stroke Association reports that 10 percent of stroke survivors make an almost complete recovery, while another 25 percent recover with only minor issues.

It's important that recovery and rehabilitation from a stroke start as soon as possible. In fact, stroke recovery should begin in the hospital.

In a hospital, a care team can stabilize your condition and assess the effects of the stroke. They can identify underlying factors and begin therapy to help you regain some of your affected skills.

Stroke recovery typically focuses on four main areas:

Speech therapy

A stroke can cause speech and language impairment. A speech and language therapist will work with you to relearn how to speak.

Or, if you find verbal communication difficult after a stroke, they'll help you find new ways of communication.

Cognitive therapy

After a stroke, many people may have changes to their thinking and reasoning skills. This can cause behavioral and mood changes.

An occupational therapist can help you work to regain your former patterns of thinking and behavior, and to manage your emotional responses.

Relearning sensory skills

If the part of your brain that relays sensory signals is affected during the stroke, you may find that your senses are "dulled" or no longer working.

That may mean that you don't feel things well, such as temperature, pressure, or pain. An occupational therapist can help you learn to adjust to this lack of sensation.

Physical therapy

Muscle tone and strength may be weakened by a stroke, and you may find you're unable to move your body as well as you could before.

A physical therapist will work with you to regain your strength and balance, and find ways to adjust to any limitations.

Rehabilitation may take place in a clinic, skilled nursing home, or your own home.

CHAPTER THREE

ANTI STROKE RECIPES

Here are some food/recipes you can take to prevent you from having stroke, and I also added some to help you when you have stroke, each of the recipes are explained by listing the ingredients alongside the preparation partern;

Almond oat bars

Ingredients

- 1/3 cup (75 mL) oat bran or wheat germ

- 1/2 cup (125 mL) almond butter

- 3 tbsp (45 mL) pure maple syrup

- 3 tbsp (45 mL) unsweetened apple sauce

- 1 1/2 cups (375 mL) large flake oats

- 1/3 cup (175 mL) dried cherries

- 1/4 cup (50 mL) sliced almonds

- 1/4 cup (50 mL) ground flaxseed

- 1/4 cup (50 mL) roasted unsalted sunflower seeds

Directions

1. Step 1

In a dry nonstick skillet, toast oat bran over medium heat for about 3 minutes or until fragrant; set aside.

2. Step 2

In a large bowl, stir together almond butter, maple syrup and apple sauce. Stir in oats, cherries, almonds, toasted oat bran, flaxseed and sunflower seeds until well combined.

3. Step 3

Pack mixture into 8 inch (1.5 L) s□uare parchment paper lined baking pan and freeze for about 2 hours or until very firm and solid. Remove from freezer and remove from pan using parchment paper as a handle. Cut into 18 bars and place in airtight container and freeze for up to 2 weeks.

Apple cranberry muffins

Ingredients

- 1 1/2 cups (375 mL) whole wheat flour

- 2 tbsp (25 mL) ground flax

- 1 tsp (5 mL) baking powder

- 1/2 tsp (2 mL) each ground cinnamon and baking soda

- 1 cup (250 mL) unsweetened applesauce

- 1/3 cup (75 mL) packed brown sugar

- 2 tbsp (25 mL) canola oil

- 1 egg

- 1 tsp (5 mL) vanilla

- 1/2 cup (125 mL) dried cranberries

Directions

1. Step 1

In a large bowl, whisk together flour, flax, baking powder, cinnamon and baking soda; set aside.

2. Step 2

In another bowl, whisk together applesauce, sugar, oil, egg and vanilla. Pour over flour mixture and stir until just combined. Stir in cranberries.

3. Step 3

Divide batter among 12 greased or paper lined muffin tins. Bake in 400° F (200° C) oven for about 12 minutes or until golden and firm when touched.

Banana maple blueberry muffins

Ingredients

- 1 cup (250 mL) chopped pitted medjool dates

- 1/2 cup (125 mL) water

- 1 cup (250 mL) cooked brown or green lentils

- 3 tbsp (45 mL) pure maple syrup

- 1 very ripe banana, peeled and mashed

- 1 egg

- 1 tsp (5 mL) vanilla

- 1 3/4 cups (425 mL) all purpose flour with added bran (nutri flour)

* 3 tbsp (45 mL) ground flax

* 1 tsp (5 mL) each ground cinnamon and baking powder

* 1/2 tsp (2 mL) baking soda

* 1/2 cup (125 mL) milk

* 1 cup (250 mL) fresh or frozen blueberries

Directions

1. Step 1

Preheat oven to 400 °F (200 °C). In a saucepan, bring dates and water to a simmer. Cover and cook for 3 minutes or until very soft.

2. Step 2

Pour date mixture into food processor with lentils and maple syrup. Blend until smooth. Scrape into a bowl and stir in mashed banana, egg and vanilla.

3. Step 3

In a large bowl, whisk together flour, flax, cinnamon, baking powder and soda. Pour date mixture over top; add milk and stir to combine. Stir in blueberries.

4. Step 4

Divide batter among 12 greased or paper lined muffin tins. Bake in 400° F (200 °C) oven for about 15 minutes or until cake tester inserted in centre comes out clean.

Avocado and egg breakfast sandwich

Ingredients

- 4 eggs

- 1/4 tsp (1.25 mL) pepper

- 1 tbsp (15 mL) olive oil

- ½ ripe avocado, peeled, pitted and sliced

- 1 tbsp (15 mL) lime juice

- 4 lettuce leaves

- 16 slices cucumber

- 1/3 cup (75 mL) sprouts

- 4 whole wheat English muffins, toasted

Directions

1. Step 1

Whisk together eggs and pepper. In non-stick skillet, heat oil over medium-low heat; pour in egg mixture. Cook, stirring constantly, until eggs are creamy and softly set, approximately 5 minutes.

2. Step 2

Toss together avocado, lime juice, and pinch each of the salt and pepper. Layer lettuce, avocado, cucumber, scrambled eggs and sprouts over bottom halves of English muffins. Cap with top halves of muffins.

Breakfast strata primavera

Ingredients

- 1 tbsp (15 mL) canola oil

- 1 large onion, diced (about 2 cups/500 mL)

- 2 cloves garlic, minced

- 1/2 bunch asparagus (about 1/2 pound/250 g), trimmed and sliced into 1-inch (2.5-cm) pieces

- 1 cup (250 mL) green peas, fresh or frozen

- Canola oil cooking spray

- 1 whole-wheat baguette or other crusty bread (8 oz/500 g), cut into 1-inch (2.5-cm) cubes (about 8 cups/2 L)

- 6 large eggs

- 10 large egg whites

- 2 cups (500 mL) nonfat milk

- 1 tbsp (15 mL) Dijon mustard

- 1/4 cup (50 mL) freshly grated Parmesan cheese, lightly packed

- 2 oz (60 g) part-skim mozzarella cheese, shredded (1/2 cup/125 mL)

- 1 large carrot, shredded (1 cup/250 mL)

- 1/4 cup (50 mL) sundried tomatoes, thinly sliced

- 1 tbsp (15 mL) chopped fresh tarragon leaves or 1 tsp/5 mL dried tarragon

- 1/2 tsp (2 mL) freshly ground black pepper

Directions

1. Step 1

In large nonstick skillet, heat canola oil over medium-high heat. Add onion and cook, stirring, until softened, about 3 minutes. Add garlic and continue to cook for 1 minute more. Add asparagus and cook, stirring occasionally, until just beginning to soften, about 1 minute. Stir in peas, remove from heat and set aside.

2. Step 2

Coat 9 x 13-inch (22 x 33-cm) baking dish with canola oil cooking spray. Arrange bread cubes over bottom. In large bowl, beat whole eggs, egg whites, milk and mustard together until blended. Add vegetable mixture, both cheeses, carrot, sun-dried tomatoes, tarragon and pepper, stirring to incorporate. Pour mixture over bread, making sure liquid saturates bread. Cover with plastic wrap and refrigerate overnight or at least 8 hours.

3. Step 3

Remove strata from refrigerator, uncover and allow to sit at room temperature while you preheat oven to 350 °F (180 °C). (Do not keep at room temperature for more than 20 minutes.) Bake until set and top forms golden brown crust, 70-80 minutes.

Buttermilk blueberry muffins

Ingredients

- 1 cup (250 mL) buttermilk

- 1 cup (250 mL) pitted prunes

- 3 tbsp (45 mL) canola oil

- 1 tsp (5 mL) vanilla

- 1 cup (250 mL) whole wheat flour

- 2 tbsp (25 mL) wheat germ

- 1 tsp (5 mL) ground ginger

- 1 1/2 tsp (7 mL) baking powder

- 3/4 tsp (4 mL) baking soda

- 1 cup (250 mL) fresh blueberries

Directions

1. Step 1

In a food processor or small food chopper, puree 3/4 cup (175 mL) of the buttermilk with prunes until prunes are in very small pieces and mixture is thickened. Pulse in oil and vanilla.

2. Step 2

In a large bowl, whisk together flour, wheat germ, ginger, baking powder and soda. Pour buttermilk mixture over top and remaining buttermilk and stir gently to combine. Fold in blueberries.

3. Step 3

Scoop batter into greased or paper lined muffins tins and bake in 375 °F (190 °C) oven for about 15 minutes or until tester inserted comes out clean.

Chocolate zucchini muffins

Ingredients

- 1 cup (250 mL) whole wheat flour

- 1/2 cup (125 mL) all purpose flour

- 1/2 cup (125 mL) wheat bran

- 1/2 cup (125 mL) unsweetened cocoa powder

- 2 tsp (10 mL) baking powder

- 1 tsp (5 mL) baking soda

- 1/4 tsp (1 mL) ground cinnamon

- 1/2 cup (125 mL) packed brown sugar

- 1/3 cup (75 mL) canola oil

- 2 eggs

- 1/2 cup (125 mL) milk

- 1 tbsp (15 mL) vanilla

- 2 cups (500 mL) grated zucchini

Directions

1. Step 1

Preheat oven to 400° F (200° C)

2. Step 2

In a large bowl whisk together whole wheat and all purpose flours, wheat bran, cocoa powder, baking powder and soda and cinnamon; set aside.

3. Step 3

In another bowl, whisk together sugar and oil until combined. Whisk in eggs one at a time; add milk and vanilla. Pour over flour mixture. Add zucchini and stir until dry ingredients are moistened.

4. Step 4

Spoon into greased or paper lined muffin pan. Bake in 400° F (200° C) oven for about 18 minutes or tester inserted in centre comes out clean.

Freezer options: Wrap each muffin individually with plastic wrap and place in airtight container for up to 1 month. Defrost at room temperature or in the microwave.

Storage: Keep in container at room temperature for up to 3 days.

Cinnamon oatmeal pancakes

Ingredients

- 2 cups (500 mL) rolled oats

- 2 1/2 cups (625 mL) buttermilk, divided

- 1/2 cup (125 mL) whole wheat flour or oat flour

- 1 tsp (5 mL) baking powder

- 1 tsp (5 mL) baking soda

- 1/4 tsp (1 mL) cinnamon

- 1/4 tsp (1 mL) salt

- 2 large eggs

- 1/4 cup (50 mL) canola oil

- 1 tbsp (15 mL) honey or maple syrup

- canola oil cooking spray or extra canola oil for cooking

Directions

1. Step 1

In large bowl, stir together oats and 2 cups (500 mL) buttermilk. Set aside for an hour or until buttermilk is absorbed and oats are soft. (To do this ahead of time, cover and refrigerate overnight.)

2. Step 2

In small bowl, stir together flour, baking powder, baking soda, cinnamon and salt. Add to softened oatmeal.

3. Step 3

Add remaining 1/2 cup (125 mL) buttermilk along with eggs, canola oil, honey or maple syrup. Stir with rubber spatula just until well combined.

4. Step 4

Heat large, heavy skillet over medium-high heat and spray with canola oil cooking spray or brush with canola oil.

5. Step 5

Cook about 1/2 cup (125 mL) batter at a time; spread it out with bottom of ladle or spoon (it will be thick) to about 4 inches (10 cm) in diameter. Turn heat down to medium-low and cook until edges appear dry and bubbles begin to break on surface. Using thin spatula, flip and cook until golden on other side.

6. Step 6

Repeat with remaining batter. If you like, keep cooked pancakes warm in 200 °F (100 °C) oven while cooking the rest.

Cranberry granola bars

Ingredients

- 1/2 cup (125 mL) chopped and pitted medjool dates

- 1 cup (250 mL) orange juice

- 1/4 cup (50 mL) soy or nut butter

- 1 tsp (5 mL) vanilla

- 1 tsp (5 mL) cinnamon

- 2 cups (500 mL) large flake oats

- 1/3 cup (75 mL) wheat germ

- 2 tbsp (25 mL) ground flaxseed

- 1/4 cup (60 mL) dried cranberries or raisins

Directions

1. Step 1

In a small saucepan, combine dates and orange juice. Bring to a gentle simmer over medium heat for about 5 minutes or until very soft. Add soy butter, vanilla and cinnamon and stir until smooth.

2. Step 2

In a large bowl, combine oats, wheat germ, flaxseed and cranberries. Pour over date mixture and stir to combine. Spread into a parchment paper lined 8 inch (1.5 L) baking pan and press down evenly.

3. Step 3

Bake in a 350 F (180 C) oven for about 25 minutes or until golden and firm to the touch. Let cool before cutting into bars.

Crepes with shrimp spinach and herb filling

Ingredients

- 1 cup (250 mL) 1% milk

- 3 large eggs

- 1/2 cup (125 mL) whole-grain pastry flour

- 1/2 cup (125 mL) all-purpose flour

- 2 tbsp (25 mL) canola oil

- Filling

- 1 tbsp (15 mL) canola oil

- 1 medium shallot, finely chopped (about 3 Tbsp/45 mL)

- 1 clove garlic, minced

- 2 tsp (10 mL) all-purpose flour

- 1/2 cup (125 mL) 1% milk

- 5 cups (1.25 L) fresh baby spinach leaves, coarsely chopped

- 1 lb (500 g) medium shrimp, peeled and deveined, tails removed

- 1/4 tsp (1 mL) freshly ground black pepper

- 1/4 cup (50 mL) fresh basil leaves, sliced into ribbons

- 2 tbsp (25 mL) fresh parsley leaves, coarsely chopped

- Canola oil cooking spray

Directions

1. Crêpes mix:

In blender, place milk and eggs and blend to combine. Add both flours and blend until very smooth, about 15 seconds. Add canola oil and blend until incorporated, 5 seconds more. Pour batter into medium bowl, cover and place in refrigerator while you prepare filling.

2. To make filling:

In large, nonstick skillet, heat canola oil over medium heat. Add shallot and cook until softened but not brown, about 2 minutes. Add garlic and cook 30 seconds more. Sprinkle flour into pan and cook, stirring until incorporated, about 30 seconds. Drizzle in milk and cook, stirring continuously until thickened, about 2 minutes. Stir in spinach and cook until it is just wilted, about 30 seconds. Add shrimp and pepper and cook, stirring once or twice, until shrimp just turn pink, about 2-3 minutes. Remove from heat and cover.

3. To make crêpes:

Heat crêpe pan or 10-inch (25-cm) nonstick skillet with 8-inch (20-cm) base over medium heat. Spray pan with canola oil cooking spray. Ladle 1/4-cup (50-mL) batter into center of pan. Tilt and rotate pan so batter forms thin layer in bottom. Cook until top is no longer li◻uid and bottom is nicely browned, about 1 minute. Flip crêpe and cook other side until light brown, about 15 seconds more. Repeat with remaining batter until you have eight crêpes. (You will not need to re-spray pan.) Stack finished crepes on plate.

To fill crêpes:

Return shrimp-spinach mixture to skillet at medium heat and cook until warmed and shrimp are cooked through, 1-2 minutes. Remove from heat and stir in herbs. Place one crêpe on plate, top with about 1/3 cup (75 mL) of shrimp mixture in center and roll up. Repeat with remaining crêpes and shrimp mixture. Serve immediately.

Bean, lentil and brown rice casserole

Ingredients

- 1 1/2 tbsp (20 mL) canola oil

- 1 cup (250 mL) chopped onion

- 3 cloves garlic, minced

- 3 tbsp (45 mL) chopped, canned chipotle peppers in adobo sauce

- 1 tsp (5 mL) dried oregano

- 1 tsp (5 mL) dried savory

- 1/2 tsp (2 mL) freshly ground black pepper

- 1 cup (250 mL) sodium-reduced medium or hot salsa

- 1 cup (250 mL) raw brown basmati rice

- 1 cup (250 mL) green lentils

- 1 can (19 oz/540 mL) kidney beans, drained and rinsed

- 4 1/2 (1.125 L) cups water

- 1 bay leaf

- 1 cup (250 mL) reduced-fat shredded cheddar cheese

Directions

1. Step 1

Preheat oven to 350 ºF (180 ºC). Lightly spray 3-Quart (3.4 L) casserole with canola oil cooking spray and set aside.

2. Step 2

In large soup pot, heat canola oil over medium-high heat. Add onions, reduce heat to medium and cook for 3-4 minutes. Add garlic, chipotle peppers, oregano, savory and black pepper and cook for 1-2 minutes more. Stir in salsa and deglaze pan.

3. Step 3

Add brown rice, lentils, kidney beans, water and bay leaf. Bring to a boil. Transfer mixture to prepared baking dish. Cover with foil and bake in preheated oven for about 1¼ -1½ hours or until rice and lentils are tender and no water remains. Stir twice during baking, replacing foil before returning to oven. Remove bay leaf before serving.

4. Step 4

Remove from oven, remove bay leaf and sprinkle with cheese. Leave foil off and return to oven for 3-4 minutes to melt cheese.

Bean, sweet potato and garlic stew

Ingredients

- 1 tbsp (15 mL) canola oil

- 1 onion, thinly sliced

- 6 cloves garlic, thinly sliced

- 2 stalks celery, thinly sliced

- 2 sweet potatoes (about 1 3/4 lb/800 g), peeled and chopped

- 1 tbsp (15 mL) chopped fresh thyme leaves

- 1/4 tsp (1 mL) pepper

- 2 cups (500 mL) sodium reduced vegetable broth

- 2 bay leaves

- 1 can (19 oz/540 mL) no salt added white kidney beans, drained and rinsed

- 1 tub (142 g) baby spinach, coarsely chopped

Directions

1. Step 1

In a large saucepan, heat oil over medium heat. Cook onion, garlic and celery for 3 minutes to soften. Stir in sweet potatoes, thyme and pepper to coat well.

2. Step 2

Add broth and bay leaves and bring to a boil. Reduce heat; cover and simmer gently for 15 minutes or until sweet potatoes are tender but firm.

3. Step 3

Uncover and stir in kidney beans and spinach and cook for 5 minutes to heat through. Remove bay leaves before serving.

Broccoli and tofu sheet pan dinner

Ingredients

- 1 head broccoli (at least 2 stalks)

- 175 g or half a 350 g pkg extra firm tofu, diced

- Half a red onion, sliced

- 2 tbsp (25 mL) sodium reduced soy sauce

- 2 tsp (10 mL) sesame oil

- 1 clove garlic, minced

- 1 tsp (5 mL) minced fresh ginger

- 1/2 tsp (2 mL) sriracha chili sauce or hot sauce (optional)

- 1 tsp (5 mL) toasted sesame seeds (optional)

Directions

1. Step 1

Cut stalks from broccoli and peel. Cut broccoli top into small florets and chop peeled broccoli stem; place in a large bowl. Add tofu and red onion.

2. Step 2

Drizzle vegetables and tofu with soy sauce and oil. Add garlic, ginger and sriracha, if using. Toss well until everything is coated.

3. Step 3

Spread onto a parchment paper lined baking sheet. Roast in 400° F (200° C) oven for about 20 minutes or until golden. Remove from oven and return to bowl.

4. Step 4

Sprinkle with sesame seeds, if using before serving.

Cauliflower tacos

Ingredients

- 1 head cauliflower, trimmed

- 1/2 cup (125 mL) no salt added vegetable broth or water

- 1 tbsp (15 mL) canola oil

- 1 small onion, finely chopped

- 2 cloves garlic, minced

- 1 cup (250 mL) grated extra firm tofu

- 1 red bell pepper, diced

- 1 tbsp (15 mL) chili powder

- 1 tsp (5 mL) each dried oregano leaves and ground cumin

- 1/4 tsp (1 mL) cayenne

- 3/4 cup (175 mL) medium salsa

- 1 pkg (156 g) hard corn taco shells (12) or 8 small whole wheat flour tortillas

- 1 cup (250 mL) shredded lettuce or coleslaw mix

- 1 small avocado, diced

- 1/2 cup (125 mL) shredded light or reduced fat old cheddar (optional)

- plain greek yogurt (optional)

Directions

1. Step 1

Cut cauliflower into quarters and remove tough inner stem. Chop remaining cauliflower into about 1/2 inch (1 cm) pieces. Place in a large nonstick skillet. Add broth and bring to a simmer. Cover and cook for 5 minutes. Uncover and pour out into a bowl.

2. Step 2

Return skillet to medium heat and add oil. Add onion and garlic; cook, stirring for 2 minutes. Add tofu, red pepper, chili powder, oregano, cumin and cayenne and cook for 2 minutes. Increase heat to medium high and return cauliflower to skillet. Cook, stirring for about 5 minutes or until cauliflower starts to brown. Stir in salsa and cook for 2 minutes to heat through.

3. Step 3

Spoon mixture among taco shells and top with lettuce, avocado and cheese, if using. Top with yogurt if desired.

Curried egg pitas

Ingredients

- 8 eggs, beaten

- 1/4 cup (60 mL) finely chopped green onion

- 1/4 cup (60 mL) finely chopped green pepper

- 1 tbsp (15 mL) canola oil

- 4 small (6-inch/15 cm) pocket-style whole-wheat pitas, halved

- 1/4 cup (60 mL) mango chutney

- 2 tsp (10 mL) ginger powder

- 2 tsp (10 mL) mild red curry paste

- 1/4 tsp (1.25 mL) black pepper

- 1/4 cup (60 mL) plain non-fat yogurt

- 1 cup (250 mL) julienne cucumber

- 1 cup (250 mL) julienne carrots

- 4 cups (1 L) lightly packed baby spinach, divided

Directions

1. Step 1

Beat eggs. Stir in the green onion and green pepper until well combined.

2. Step 2

Heat oil in large non-stick skillet set over medium heat. Pour egg mixture into pan. Cook, without stirring, for 2 minutes or until eggs are just set.

3. Step 3

Meanwhile, cut each pita in half and open the pockets. Blend mango chutney, ginger powder, curry paste and pepper with yogurt, until well combined.

4. Step 4

Inside each halved pita, spread an e□ual amount of sauce. Divide the cucumber, carrots, spinach and egg mixture evenly between the pockets. Serve immediately.

Curried lentils and vegetables

Ingredients

- 2 tbsp (25 mL) canola oil

- 1 medium onion, minced

- 2 cloves garlic, minced

- 2 tsp (10 mL) curry powder

- 1 tsp (5 mL) ground cinnamon

- ½ tsp (2 mL) ground cloves

- ½ tsp (2 mL) dried thyme

- 1 cup (250 mL) water

- ½ cup (125 mL) dried green lentils, rinsed

- 1 cup (250 mL) carrots, peeled and diced

- 1 medium sweet potato, peeled and cubed

- 1 (14 oz / 398 mL) can low sodium diced tomatoes

- 1 tbsp (15 mL) cooking sherry

- ¼ tsp (1 mL) freshly ground pepper

- Chopped cilantro, optional garnish

Directions

1. Step 1

In large saucepan with lid, heat canola oil to medium heat. Add onion and sauté until softened, about 5 minutes. Add garlic, curry powder, cinnamon, cloves and thyme. Stir and cook for about 2 minutes.

2. Step 2

Add water, lentils, carrots, sweet potato, tomatoes (and their li□uid) and sherry. Simmer for about 15 minutes or until vegetables are tender.

3. Step 3

Season to taste with pepper and garnish with cilantro, if using. Serve.

Egg and pepper skillet supper

Ingredients

- 2 tsp (10 mL) canola oil

- 3 peppers, one red, yellow and orange or green, thinly sliced

- 1 1/2 tsp (7 mL) dried oregano leaves

- 1 tub (5 oz/142 g) baby spinach

- 3 cloves garlic, minced

- 1/4 tsp (1 mL) hot pepper flakes

- 4 eggs

- 1/4 cup (50 mL) chunky salsa

Directions

1. Step 1

In a large nonstick skillet, heat oil over medium high heat. Add red, yellow and green peppers and oregano and saute for 5 minutes or until starting to brown. Reduce heat to medium and stir in spinach, garlic and hot pepper flakes; cook stirring for about 3 minutes or until spinach is wilted.

2. Step 2

Make 4 little holes in the pepper mixture and crack an egg into each hole. Cover and cook for about 2 minutes or until egg is set or until desired doneness. Remove from heat and using flat spatula, lift out egg and pepper mixture onto 4 plates. Top with salsa to serve.

Eggplant lentil curry

Ingredients

- 2 tsp (10 mL) canola oil

- 1 onion, chopped

- 3 cloves garlic, minced

- 1 tbsp (15 mL) minced fresh ginger

- 2 Asian eggplants about 12 oz/375 g, chopped

- 1 tbsp (15 mL) curry powder

- 1/2 tsp (2 mL) cumin seeds

- 1 1/2 cups (375 mL) sodium reduced vegetable broth

- 1 can (19 oz/540 mL) no salt added lentils, drained and rinsed

- 1 tomato, chopped

- 1/2 cup fresh cilantro leaves, chopped

- 1/2 tsp (2 mL) hot pepper sauce (optional)

Directions

1. Step 1

In a saucepan, heat oil over medium heat and cook onion, garlic and ginger for 3 minutes or until softened.

2. Step 2

Stir in eggplant, curry powder and cumin, sauté for 1 minute.

3. Step 3

Add broth, lentils and tomato; bring to a simmer.

4. Step 4

Cook, stirring occasionally about 15 minutes or until eggplant is very tender. Stir in cilantro to serve.

Fusilli pasta with chile sauce and black bean fennel relish

Ingredients

- 8 dried New Mexican chiles

- Boiling water, as needed

- 1 cup (250 mL) fire-roasted tomatoes, drained

- 1 cup (250 mL) black beans, drained and rinsed

- 1 tbsp (15 mL) canola oil

- 10 oz (300 g) whole-grain fusilli pasta or other spiral-shaped pasta

- 1 small zucchini, grated

- 1 small fennel bulb, cut in half, cored and thinly sliced

- 2 tbsp (25 mL) finely chopped parsley

- 2 scallions, thinly sliced

- 1 lemon, zested and juiced

- 1 1/2 cups (375 mL) black beans, drained and rinsed

- 1 tbsp (15 mL) canola oil

- 1/4 cup (50 mL) feta cheese for garnish

Directions

1. Step 1

To prepare chile sauce: In bowl, place chiles and cover with boiling water to rehydrate. Cover bowl with plastic wrap and let chiles sit 30 minutes.

When chiles have rehydrated, remove from water, reserving 1 cup (250 mL) chile water for later use. Make slit down each chile, split them lengthwise and remove seeds. Be careful not to touch your eyes or other sensitive areas while handling chiles. Once completed, wash hands thoroughly.

2. Step 2

In food processor, add chiles, 1 cup (250 mL) reserved chile water, tomatoes, 1 cup (250 mL) black beans and canola oil. Purée until mixture is smooth and reserve for later use.

3. Step 3

Cook pasta according to package instructions. Drain pasta in colander but do not rinse with water.

4. Step 4

To prepare black bean relish: In bowl, combine zucchini, fennel, parsley, scallions, lemon, remaining black beans and canola oil. Set aside.

5. Step 5

In large saucepan, warm chile sauce over medium-low heat, stirring occasionally, 3-5 minutes, until heated. Remove from heat; add pasta and stir briefly to coat noodles with sauce.

6. Step 6

Transfer pasta to large serving bowl and add black bean-fennel relish to center of pasta. Garnish with feta cheese and serve.

Grilled veggie and grain platter

Ingredients

- 1/2 cup (125 mL) quinoa

- 1 cup (250 mL) sodium reduced vegetable broth

- 1 small clove garlic, minced

- 2 tbsp (25 mL) chopped fresh basil

- 1 zucchini, sliced or 1 cup (250 mL) chopped asparagus

- 1 small head radicchio, chopped

- 1 small yellow or red bell pepper, chopped

- 2 tbsp (25 mL) chopped fresh parsley

- 2 tsp (10 mL) canola oil

- 1/4 tsp (1 mL) pepper

- 3 tbsp (45 mL) balsamic vinegar

Directions

1. Step 1

In a small saucepan, bring □uinoa, broth and garlic to a boil. Reduce heat to low, cover and cook for about 15 minutes or until broth is absorbed. Stir in basil; set aside.

2. Step 2

Meanwhile, toss zucchini, radicchio, yellow pepper, parsley, oil and pepper together in grill basket. Place on medium high grill, stirring occasionally for about 10 minutes or until vegetables are charred slightly and softened.

3. Step 3

Spread □uinoa onto large serving platter and top with vegetables. Drizzle all over with balsamic vinegar to serve.

Italian spinach baked eggs and noodles

Ingredients

- 2 tsp (10 mL) extra virgin olive oil

- 1 shallot, finely chopped

- 2 cloves garlic, minced

- 2 tsp (10 mL) dried oregano leaves

- 1/4 tsp (1 mL) hot pepper flakes

- 1 bottle (700 mL) passata (strained tomatoes)

- 1 pkg (5 oz/142 g) baby spinach, chopped

- 1 yellow or orange bell pepper, diced

- 4 eggs

- 1/4 tsp (1 mL) fresh ground pepper

- 3 tbsp (45 mL) fresh grated Parmesan

- 3 cups (750 mL) egg white broad pasta noodles

Directions

1. Step 1

In a large ovenproof nonstick skillet, heat oil over medium heat and cook shallot, garlic, oregano and hot pepper flakes. Pour in passata and bring to a boil. Reduce heat and simmer for 5 minutes.

2. Step 2

Stir in spinach and pepper; cook for 5 minutes or until wilted.

3. Step 3

Crack eggs, one at a time into a small bowl and slip eggs into simmering sauce. Sprinkle with ground pepper. Place in preheated 400 F (200 C) oven for about 10 minutes or until eggs set or cooked to desired doneness.

4. Step 4

Meanwhile, in a pot of boiling water, cook noodles for about 8 minutes or until tender but firm. Drain well and keep warm.

5. Step 5

Sprinkle eggs with cheese and spoon with sauce over top of noodles to serve.

Indonesian tofu stew with spring vegetables

Ingredients

- 1 tbsp (15 mL) freshly grated ginger

- Juice of one medium sized lime

- 1 1/2 tbsp (20 mL) canola oil, divided

- 1 (12 oz / 350 g) block of firm or extra firm tofu, diced into cubes

- 1 large onion, diced

- 2 cloves garlic, minced

- 1 tsp (5 mL) ground cumin

- 1 tsp (5 mL) ground coriander

- 1/4 tsp (1 mL) ground cloves

- 1 cup (250 mL) sodium-reduced vegetable or chicken broth

- 1 cup (250 mL) light coconut milk L

- 2 cups (500 mL) green beans, cut in 2 inch (5 cm) pieces

- 1 red bell pepper, diced

- 1 medium zucchini, diced

- 2 tbsp (25 mL) fresh cilantro

Directions

1. Step 1

In a bowl, marinate tofu with the ginger, lime juice and 1/2 tbsp (7 mL) canola oil. Toss well to coat. This can be done about 30 minutes ahead of time and up to overnight in the refrigerator.

2. Step 2

In a large saucepan, no lid re□uired heat remaining 1 tbsp (15 mL) canola oil. Add onion and cook for about 6 minutes or until softened and slightly browned. Add garlic, cumin, coriander and cloves and stir for 2 minutes.

3. Step 3

To saucepan, add stock and coconut milk. Simmer, uncovered, for about 10 minutes until slightly thickened.

4. Step 4

Add green beans, bell pepper and zucchini and cook for about 10 minutes more or until vegetables are tender. Add marinated tofu and cook an additional 5 minutes. Garnish with cilantro. Serve over steamed brown rice or ꠱uinoa, if desired.

Blackened basa fillets with ratatouille

Ingredients

- Ratatouille:

- 1 tbsp (15 mL) canola oil, divided

- 1 1/2 cups (375 mL) eggplant, diced

- 1 cup (250 mL) zucchini, diced

- 1 3/4 cups (425 mL) tomatoes, diced

- 2/3 cup (150 mL) each: diced sweet red pepper and diced red onion

- 1 clove garlic, minced

- 1 tsp (5 mL) dried basil (or 1 tbsp (15 mL) chopped fresh basil)

- Basa:

- 1 tsp (5 mL) each: pepper, onion powder and paprika

- 1/2 tsp (2 mL) dried thyme

- 1/4 tsp (1 mL) each: garlic powder and cumin

- Pinch cayenne pepper

- 1 (200 g) basa fillet

Directions

1. Step 1

In Dutch oven over medium heat, heat 1 tsp (5 mL) of the canola oil. Add eggplant, zucchini, tomatoes, red pepper, onion, garlic and basil. Cook, covered, for 12 minutes, stirring occasionally.

2. Step 2

Meanwhile in small bowl mix together spices. Brush basa fillet with 1 tsp (5 mL) of the canola oil. Sprinkle spice mixture over both sides of fish.

3. Step 3

Heat remaining canola oil in large non-stick skillet over medium-high heat. Cook fish 2 to 3 minutes per side until the fish flakes easily.

4. Step 4

Spoon half of the ratatouille onto each plate. Divide fish in half; place over ratatouille.

Cod fish with potatoes, fennel and carrots

Ingredients

- 2 tbsp (25 mL) canola oil

- 1 medium onion, thinly sliced

- 2 cloves garlic, minced

- 1 small fennel bulb, trimmed and cut into thin slices, a few fronds reserved

- 4 small potatoes, thinly sliced

- 2 large carrots, peeled and shaved into large pieces

- 3/4 cup (175 mL) low-sodium chicken broth

- 2 Tbsp (25 mL) tomato paste

- 3 wide strips orange peel, white pith removed

- 4 cod fish fillets (4 oz/125 g each)

Directions

1. Step 1

In large non-stick pan, heat canola oil over medium-high heat. Add onion and garlic and sauté until onion is soft, about 6 to 7 minutes. Add fennel and continue to cook until fennel is tender crisp, about 4 to 5 minutes. Add potatoes and carrots. Continue cooking.

2. Step 2

Whisk together chicken broth and tomato paste and add to pan along with orange peel. Simmer 10 minutes, covered.

3. Step 3

Place cod fillets on top of vegetables. Cover pan and cook 10 minutes longer or until fish is cooked throughout. To serve, garnish with fennel fronds.

Creamy clam chowder recipe

Ingredients

- 2 tsp (10 mL) canola oil

- 1 pkg (8 oz/227 g) mushrooms, chopped

- 1 small onion, diced

- 3 cloves garlic, minced

- 2 stalks celery, diced

- 2 tbsp (25 mL) chopped fresh parsley or 1 tbsp (15 mL) dried parsley

- 1 tbsp (15 mL) chopped fresh tarragon or 1 tsp (5 mL) dried tarragon

- 3 tbsp (45 mL) all purpose flour

- 2 cups (500 mL) skim milk

- 1 cup (250 mL) sodium reduced vegetable or fish broth

- 1 can (142 g) baby clams, drained and rinsed

- 1 cup (250 mL) corn kernels

Directions

1. Step 1

In a soup pot, heat oil over medium heat and cook mushrooms, onion, garlic, celery, parsley and tarragon for about 8 minutes or until liquid starts to evaporate. Stir in flour until well coated.

2. Step 2

Pour in milk and broth; bring to a gentle boil. Stir in clams and corn and simmer gently for about 5 minutes or until thickened and bubbling slightly.

Corn sweet potato and salmon chowder

Ingredients

- 2 tsp (10 mL) vegetable oil

- 1 onion, finely chopped

- 1 clove garlic, minced

- 1 tsp (5 mL) dried dill weed

- Pepper

- 1 sweet potato, peeled if desired and cut into 1/2-inch (1 cm) cubes (about 2 cups/500 mL)

- 1 1/2 cup (375 mL) corn kernels (fresh or frozen, thawed)

- 2 cups (500 mL) water

- 1/4 cup (50 mL) all-purpose flour

- 2 cups (500 mL) 1% milk

- 12 oz (375 g) skinless salmon fillet, cut into chunks

- 1 tsp (5 mL) grated lemon zest

- 3 tbsp (45 mL) freshly squeezed lemon juice

Directions

1. Step 1

In a large pot, heat oil over medium heat. Sauté onion, garlic, dill and 1/4 tsp (1 mL) pepper for about 5 minutes or until onions are softened. Stir in potatoes, corn and water; bring to a boil over high heat. Cover, reduce heat to medium-low and simmer for 5 to 10 minutes or until potatoes are almost tender.

2. Step 2

Increase heat to medium. Whisk flour into milk and gradually stir into pot. Stir in salmon. Simmer, uncovered and stirring often but gently, for about 5 minutes or until salmon is firm and opaque and soup is thickened (do not let boil). Stir in lemon zest and juice and season to taste with pepper. Ladle into warmed bowls.

Crunchy salmon sticks

Ingredients

- 1 lb (500 g) centre cut salmon fillet, skinned

- 1 egg white, lightly beaten

- 1 tsp (5 mL) Dijon mustard

- 1 tsp (5 mL) chopped fresh thyme or 2 mL (1/2 tsp) dried thyme leaves

- 1 cup (250 mL) finely crushed bran or cornflakes

- 2 tsp (10 mL) chili powder

- 1 tsp (5 mL) paprika

- 1/4 tsp (1 mL) cayenne pepper

Directions

1. Step 1

Preheat oven to 425 ⬚F (220 ° C)

2. Step 2

Cut salmon into 8 equal strips and set aside.

3. Step 3

In shallow dish, whisk together egg white, mustard and thyme.

4. Step 4

In another shallow dish, stir together bran flakes, chili powder, paprika and cayenne pepper. Dip salmon in egg, letting excess drip off. Coat in bran flake mixture and place on parchment paper lined baking sheet.

5. Step 5

Bake in 425☐ F (220° C) oven for about 10 minutes or until golden and flakes when tested with fork.

Grilled scallops puttanesca

Ingredients

- 12 sea scallops

- 1 tbsp (15 mL) lemon juice

- 1 tsp (5 mL) chopped fresh thyme

- 1 clove garlic, rasped

- 2 red peppers, ☐uartered

- 2 tsp (10 mL) extra virgin olive oil

- 1 cup (250 mL) halved grape tomatoes

- 2 tsp (10 mL) capers, chopped

- 1 clove garlic, minced

- 1/4 tsp (1 mL) hot pepper flakes

- 1 tbsp (15 mL) red wine vinegar

Directions

1. Step 1

In a bowl, coat scallops with lemon juice, thyme and garlic; set aside.

2. Step 2

Spray peppers with cooking spray and grill over medium high heat for about 8 minutes, turning occasionally until tender and golden. Remove to cutting board and chop; set aside.

3. Step 3

In a skillet, heat oil over medium high heat and saute tomatoes, capers, garlic and hot pepper flakes for 2 minutes. Stir in chopped peppers and vinegar. Stir to combine; remove from heat.

4. Step 4

Spray scallops with cooking spray and place on grill over medium high heat and grill, turning once for about 4 minutes or until grill marked and opaⓆue. Serve on tomato and pepper mixture.

Ginger shrimp with gai lan

Ingredients

• 5 large dry shiitake mushrooms, soaked in water and sliced

• 1 1/2 tbsp (20 mL) canola oil

• 1/2 lb (250 g) large uncooked shrimp

• 1 medium onion, cut into wedges

• 1 clove garlic, minced

• 5 large stalks gai lan (Chinese broccoli), cut into medium size pieces

• 1 tbsp (15 mL) fresh ginger

• 1/8 tsp (0.5 mL) five spice powder

• 1 tbsp (15 mL) sweet chili sauce

- 1 tbsp (15 mL) cornstarch

- 1 cup (250 mL) low sodium chicken broth

- 1/4 cup (50 mL) cashew nuts, coarsely chopped

Directions

1. Step 1

Soak mushrooms in water for about 30 minutes.

2. Step 2

Pour canola oil into a large wok and heat over medium high heat. Quickly stir fry shrimp until just cooked. Remove from wok. Add a bit more canola oil if necessary. Add onion, garlic, gai lan stalks (leave out leafy parts until the end of cooking time), ginger, five spice powder, and sweet chili sauce. Stir fry for 3-4 minutes to cook vegetables.

3. Step 3

Dissolve corn starch in broth and add to vegetables. Heat mixture for 1 minute.

4. Step 4

Add shrimp and gai lan leaves to the mixture and heat through. Garnish with cashew nuts and serve immediately.

Grilled shrimp skewers

Ingredients

- 2 tsp (10 mL) rasped fresh ginger

- 2 cloves garlic, rasped

- 2 tbsp (30 mL) sodium reduced soy sauce

- 1/4 tsp (1 mL) sriracha sauce (or 1/2 tsp/2 mL for a spicier kick)

- 1 pkg (454 g) large raw shrimp, thawed peeled and deveined

- 2 tbsp (25 mL) chopped fresh cilantro (optional)

- 2 cups (500 mL) baby arugula

Directions

1. Step 1

In a bowl, whisk together ginger, garlic, soy sauce and sriracha. Add shrimp and toss to coat evenly. Let stand 10 minutes.

2. Step 2

Using small skewers, push 2 shrimps onto each skewer and spray lightly with cooking spray.

3. Step 3

Place shrimp on grill over medium heat and grill shrimp turning once for about 5 minutes or until cooked through. Garnish with cilantro if desired. Serve on arugula.

Grilled tortilla and shrimp salad

Ingredients

*   1 bag (454 g) frozen jumbo shrimp, thawed, peeled and deveined

*   2 tsp (10 mL) smoked paprika

*   1 tsp (5 mL) canola oil

*   1 clove garlic, minced

- 4 small whole wheat or corn tortillas

- 2 tbsp (25 mL) chopped fresh cilantro

- 1 tbsp (15 mL) lemon juice

- 5 cups (1.25 L) mixed spring greens

- 2 tbsp (25 mL) sherry vinegar

- Pinch fresh ground pepper

- 1 cup (250 mL) halved grape tomatoes

Directions

1. Step 1

In a bowl, toss shrimp with paprika, oil and pepper. Place on oiled grill over medium high heat, turning once for about 4 minutes or until firm and pink. Remove to a clean bowl and toss with cilantro and lemon juice.

2. Step 2

Place tortillas on grill and toast on both sides. Place one on each dinner plate.

3. Step 3

In another bowl, toss greens with vinegar and pepper. Top each tortilla with greens and sprinkle with tomatoes. Top with grilled shrimp to serve.

Halibut en papillote

Ingredients

- 1 tbsp (15 mL) canola oil

- 1 small yellow onion, finely diced

- 2 sprigs fresh thyme

- 2 cloves garlic, minced

- 1/2 cup (125 mL) dry white wine

- 1 jar (16 oz/455 mL) diced, fire-roasted tomatoes with juice

- 1 jar (8 oz/227 mL) artichokes, coarsely chopped

- parchment paper

- 4 halibut fillets, 4 oz/125 g each

- 1/2 tsp (2 mL) fresh ground black pepper

- Garnish

- 1 lemon, cut into quarters

- 2 tbsp (25 mL) chopped parsley

Directions

1. Step 1

In large skillet, heat canola oil to medium heat. Sauté onions with fresh thyme until soft and translucent, about 3 minutes. Add garlic; cook 1 more minute. Pour in white wine, bring to a boil and cook until almost evaporated. Add tomatoes and simmer for 20 minutes. Stir in artichokes. Remove skillet from heat, remove thyme sprigs and let cool.

2. Step 2

Preheat oven to 450 ºF (230 ºC). Cut four large rectangles of parchment paper (13 x 18 inches/33 x 46 cm each).

3. Step 3

Divide tomato-artichoke ragout among parchment paper pieces. Season each halibut fillet on both sides with pepper and place on top of ragout.

4. Step 4

Put a few drops of canola oil on top half of each parchment piece and rub it around so fish doesn't stick to it. Fold parchment over fish like book. Start sealing at edge of fold. Working in 2 inch (5 cm) sections, fold about 1/4 inch (0.5 cm) of open edges over and crease tightly. Fold again. Continue working around open edges of parchment, overlapping folded sections slightly. Finish with double fold at end of packet. Make sure folds are creased tightly so they don't open. Repeat to make three more packets.

5. Step 5

Place packets on large baking sheet. Bake in preheated oven for 10 to 12 minutes or until fish is opaque. Tear an "X" in top of packet and sprinkle with chopped parsley and juice from 1/4 lemon. Serve immediately.

Lemon flax and parsley salmon

Ingredients

- 2 tbsp (25 mL) ground flax (flax meal)

- 1 tbsp (15 mL) chopped fresh parsley

- 1 tsp (5 mL) grated lemon zest

- 1/2 tsp (2 mL) chili powder

- 4 boneless skinless salmon portions (about 4 oz/125 g each)

- 1 tsp (5 mL) canola oil

- Lemon wedges (optional)

Directions

1. Step 1

In a small bowl, stir together flax, parsley, lemon zest and chili powder; set aside.

2. Step 2

Place salmon portions onto parchment paper lined baking sheet. Brush salmon with oil and sprinkle tops with flax mixture. Press flax mixture gently on top to help stick.

3. Step 3

Roast in preheated 425F (220 C) for about 12 minutes or until fish flakes when tested with fork.

4. Step 4

Serve with lemon wedges, if desired.

Lettuce fish tacos

Ingredients

- 1 tsp (5 mL) canola oil

- 1/2 tsp (2 mL) chili powder

- Pinch cayenne pepper (optional)

- 8 oz (227 g) haddock loins or fillets

- 2 small yellow fleshed potatoes (about 8 oz/227 g)

- 2 large Boston lettuce leaves

- Half red bell pepper, thinly sliced

- 1/4 cup (50 mL) shredded carrot

- 1 tbsp (15 mL) chopped fresh parsley

- 2 lime wedges

- 2 tbsp (25 mL) 0% plain Greek yogurt

- Chopped fresh chives (optional)

Directions

1. Step 1

In a small bowl, stir together oil and chili powder. Toss haddock with oil mixture to coat and place on small baking sheet. Bake in 425° F (220° C) oven for about 10 minutes or until fish flakes when tested.

2. Step 2

Meanwhile, prick potatoes all around with a fork. Microwave for about 5 minutes or until fork tender. Let cool slightly.

3. Step 3

Wrap haddock in lettuce and sprinkle with red pepper, carrot and parsley. S ueeze lime wedge over top. Serve with potato cut in half and topped with yogurt and chives, if using.

Mahi mahi with pineapple salsa

Ingredients

- 1 1/2 cup (375 mL) diced fresh pineapple

- 1/4 cup (50 mL) chopped red onion

- 1/2 cup (125 mL) diced, seeded red bell pepper

- 1 tbsp (15 mL) chopped fresh mint

- 1 tbsp (15 mL) fresh lime juice

- 1 tbsp (15 mL) canola oil

- 4 (6 oz/170 g each) mahi-mahi fillets

- 1/4 tsp (1 mL) freshly ground pepper

Directions

1. Step 1

In bowl, combine pineapple, onion, red pepper, mint and lime juice; refrigerate until ready to serve.

2. Step 2

In nonstick skillet, heat canola oil over medium heat. Add fish and sprinkle with pepper. Cook 3-5 minutes. Turn and cook additional 3-5 minutes or until desired doneness.

3. Step 3

Top fish with pineapple salsa and serve.

One pan lemon pepper fish and veggies

Ingredients

- 8 oz (227 g) brussel sprouts, trimmed and halved

- 1 large red bell pepper, chopped

- 1 onion, sliced

- 2 cloves garlic, minced and divided

- 2 tbsp (25 mL) chopped fresh parsley, divided

- 1 tbsp (15 mL) canola oil

- 1 tsp (5 mL) Italian herb seasoning

- 2 tilapia fillets (about 8 oz/250 g)

- 1 lemon

- 1/4 tsp (1 mL) fresh ground pepper

Directions

1. Step 1

In a large bowl, toss together Brussel sprouts, pepper, onion and half each of the minced garlic and parsley. Drizzle with oil and Italian seasoning; toss again. Spread onto parchment paper lined baking sheet. Roast in 425° F (220° C) oven for 15 minutes.

2. Step 2

Zest lemon and sprinkle rind all over tilapia fillets. Sprinkle with pepper and remaining parsley and garlic. Add fillets to baking sheet and return to oven for about 12 minutes or until vegetables are golden and fish flakes when tested.

3. Step 3

Cut lemon in half and s□ueeze over fish and veggies to serve.

Panko-crusted fish sticks

Ingredients

- Edamame salsa:

- 1 1/2 cups (375 mL) frozen shelled edamame, thawed

- 1/2 medium red pepper, diced

- 1/2 small red onion, diced

- 2 tbsp (25 mL) chopped fresh cilantro

- 2 tbsp (25 mL) fresh lime juice

- 1 tbsp (15 mL) canola oil

- Fish sticks:

- 1 cup (250 mL) whole wheat panko breadcrumbs

- 1/2 tsp (2 mL) paprika

- 1/4 cup (50 mL) finely chopped walnuts

- 1/2 cup (125 mL) all-purpose or whole-wheat flour

- 4 egg whites, lightly beaten

- 1 tbsp (15 mL) canola oil

- 1 1/2 lb (750 g) grouper or cod, cut into 1 ¼ inch (3 cm) slices

- 1/2 tsp (2 mL) freshly ground black pepper

- 2 tbsp (25 mL) Dijon mustard

Directions

1. Step 1

To make edamame salsa, in medium bowl, combine edamame, red pepper, onion, cilantro, lime juice and canola oil, mixing well. Cover and chill until ready to serve.

2. Step 2

Preheat oven to 400 °F (200 °C).

3. Step 3

In shallow dish, combine panko, paprika and walnuts. In another small dish, place flour. Whisk together egg whites and canola oil in third dish.

4. Step 4

Season fish with pepper and brush with Dijon mustard. Dip fish in flour, then egg and canola oil, and dredge in panko mixture, pressing firmly to coat. Place fish on lightly oiled baking sheet. Bake for 12 to 15 minutes or until fish flakes evenly when tested with fork. Serve with Edamame Salsa.

CONCLUSION

If you suspect you may be experiencing symptoms of a stroke, it's vital that you seek emergency medical treatment as soon as possible.

Clot-busting medication can only be provided in the first hours after the signs of a stroke begin. Early treatment is one of the most effective ways to reduce your risk of long-term complications and disability.

While it's not always possible to completely prevent a stroke, certain lifestyle changes can greatly reduce your risk. Medications can also help reduce the risk of blood clots, which can lead to stroke.

If your doctor believes you might be at risk for a stroke, they will work with you to find a prevention strategy that works for you, including medical intervention and lifestyle changes.